Importan

JANUARY

....
....
....
....

MARCH

....
....
....
....

APRIL

....
....
....
....

MAY

....
....
....
....

JUNE

....
....
....
....

JULY

....
....
....
....

AUGUST

....
....
....
....

SEPTEMBER

....
....
....
....

OCTOBER

....
....
....
....

NOVEMBER

....
....
....
....

DECEMBER

....
....
....
....

January 2021

SUNDAY	MONDAY	TUESDAY
3	4	
10	11	
17	18	
24	25	
31		

WEDNESDAY	THURSDAY	FRIDAY	SATURDAY
		1	2
6	7	8	9
13	14	15	16
20	21	22	23
27	28	29	30

January 2021

AT A GLANCE

January Goals:

....
....
....

January Birthdays:

....
....
....

January Anniversaries:

....
....
....

January To Do:

☐ ....
☐ ....
☐ ....
☐ ....
☐ ....
☐ ....
☐ ....
☐ ....
☐ ....

Habit Tracker

Habit	1	2	3	4	5	6	7	8	9	10	11	12

GRATITUDE:

SHOPPING LIST:

BUDGET:

Notes:

15	16	17	18	19	20	21	22	23	24	25	26	27	28	29	30	31

January 2021

MONDAY, 28

-
-
-
-

WORKOUT:

TUESDAY, 29

-
-
-
-

WORKOUT:

WEDNESDAY, 30

-
-
-
-

WORKOUT:

THURSDAY, 31

-
-
-
-

WORKOUT:

HAPPY + HEALTHY INTENTION:

....

- ....
- ....
- ....
- ....

WORKOUT:

....

....

....

....

FRIDAY, 1

- ....
- ....
- ....

WORKOUT:

....

....

....

SATURDAY, 2

- ....
- ....
- ....

WORKOUT:

....

....

....

SUNDAY, 3

Weekly Eats:

....

....

....

....

....

To Do:

....

....

....

....

....

January 2021

MONDAY, 4

- ....
- ....
- ....
- ....

WORKOUT:

TUESDAY, 5

- ....
- ....
- ....
- ....

WORKOUT:

WEDNESDAY, 6

- ....
- ....
- ....
- ....

WORKOUT:

THURSDAY, 7

- ....
- ....
- ....
- ....

WORKOUT:

HAPPY + HEALTHY INTENTION:

....

- ....
- ....
- ....
- ....

WORKOUT:

....

....

....

FRIDAY, 8

- ....
- ....
- ....

WORKOUT:

....

....

....

SATURDAY, 9

- ....
- ....
- ....

WORKOUT:

....

....

....

SUNDAY, 10

Weekly Eats:

....

....

....

....

....

To Do:

....

....

....

....

....

January 2021

MONDAY, 11

- ....
- ....
- ....
- ....

WORKOUT:

....

....

....

....

TUESDAY, 12

- ....
- ....
- ....
- ....

WORKOUT:

....

....

....

....

WEDNESDAY, 13

- ....
- ....
- ....
- ....

WORKOUT:

....

....

....

....

THURSDAY, 14

- ....
- ....
- ....
- ....

WORKOUT:

....

....

....

....

HAPPY + HEALTHY INTENTION:

....

- ....

WORKOUT:

....

....

....

....

FRIDAY, 15

- ....
- ....
- ....

WORKOUT:

....

....

....

SATURDAY, 16

- ....
- ....
- ....

WORKOUT:

....

....

....

SUNDAY, 17

- ....
- ....
- ....

Weekly Eats

....

....

....

....

....

To Do

....

....

....

....

....

January 2021

MONDAY, 18

- ....
- ....
- ....
- ....

WORKOUT:

....
....
....

TUESDAY, 19

- ....
- ....
- ....
- ....

WORKOUT:

....
....
....

WEDNESDAY, 20

- ....
- ....
- ....
- ....

WORKOUT:

....
....
....

THURSDAY, 21

- ....
- ....
- ....

WORKOUT:

....
....
....

HAPPY + HEALTHY INTENTION:

....

FRIDAY, 22

WORKOUT:

- ....
- ....
- ....
- ....

SATURDAY, 23

WORKOUT:

- ....
- ....
- ....

SUNDAY, 24

WORKOUT:

- ....
- ....
- ....

Weekly Eats:

....

....

....

....

To Do:

....

....

....

....

January 2021

MONDAY, 25

- ....
- ....
- ....
- ....

WORKOUT:

....
....
....
....

TUESDAY, 26

- ....
- ....
- ....
- ....

WORKOUT:

....
....
....
....

WEDNESDAY, 27

- ....
- ....
- ....
- ....

WORKOUT:

....
....
....
....

THURSDAY, 28

- ....
- ....
- ....
- ....

WORKOUT:

....
....
....
....

HAPPY + HEALTHY INTENTION:

....

- ....
- ....
- ....
- ....

WORKOUT:

....
....
....
....

FRIDAY, 29

- ....
- ....
- ....

WORKOUT:

....
....
....

SATURDAY, 30

- ....
- ....
- ....

WORKOUT:

....
....
....

SUNDAY, 31

Weekly Eats:

....
....
....
....
....

To Do:

....
....
....
....
....

February 2021

SUNDAY	MONDAY	TUESDAY
	1	
7	8	
14	15	1
21	22	2
28		

EDNESDAY	THURSDAY	FRIDAY	SATURDAY
3	4	5	6
10	11	12	13
17	18	19	20
24	25	26	27

February 2021

AT A GLANCE

February Goals:

....

....

....

February Birthdays:

....

....

....

February Anniversaries:

....

....

....

February To Do:

☐ ....

☐ ....

☐ ....

☐ ....

☐ ....

☐ ....

☐ ....

☐ ....

☐ ....

Habit Tracker

Habit	1	2	3	4	5	6	7	8	9

GRATITUDE:

SHOPPING LIST:

BUDGET:

Notes:

12	13	14	15	16	17	18	19	20	21	22	23	24	25	26	27	28

February 2021

MONDAY, 1

- ....
- ....
- ....
- ....

WORKOUT:

TUESDAY, 2

- ....
- ....
- ....
- ....

WORKOUT:

WEDNESDAY, 3

- ....
- ....
- ....
- ....

WORKOUT:

THURSDAY, 4

- ....
- ....
- ....
- ....

WORKOUT:

HAPPY + HEALTHY INTENTION:

....

WORKOUT:

FRIDAY, 5

WORKOUT:

SATURDAY, 6

WORKOUT:

SUNDAY, 7

Weekly Eats

To Do:

February 2021

MONDAY, 8

- ....
- ....
- ....
- ....

WORKOUT:

- ....
- ....
- ....
- ....

TUESDAY, 9

- ....
- ....
- ....
- ....

WORKOUT:

- ....
- ....
- ....
- ....

WEDNESDAY, 10

- ....
- ....
- ....
- ....

WORKOUT:

- ....
- ....
- ....
- ....

THURSDAY, 11

- ....
- ....
- ....
- ....

WORKOUT:

- ....
- ....
- ....
- ....

....

	WORKOUT:	
•	....	**FRIDAY, 12**
•	....	
•	....	
•	....	

	WORKOUT:	
•	....	**SATURDAY, 13**
•	....	
•	....	

	WORKOUT:	
•	....	**SUNDAY, 14**
•	....	
•	....	

Weekly Eats:

....

....

....

....

....

To Do:

....

....

....

....

....

February 2021

MONDAY, 15

- ....
- ....
- ....
- ....

WORKOUT:

....
....
....

TUESDAY, 16

- ....
- ....
- ....
- ....

WORKOUT:

....
....
....

WEDNESDAY, 17

- ....
- ....
- ....
- ....

WORKOUT:

....
....
....

THURSDAY, 18

- ....
- ....
- ....
- ....

WORKOUT:

....
....
....

....

FRIDAY, 19

WORKOUT:

....

....

....

....

SATURDAY, 20

WORKOUT:

....

....

....

....

SUNDAY, 21

WORKOUT:

....

....

....

....

Weekly Eats

....

....

....

....

To Do:

....

....

....

....

February 2021

MONDAY, 22

- ....
- ....
- ....
- ....

WORKOUT:

....
....
....
....

TUESDAY, 23

- ....
- ....
- ....
- ....

WORKOUT:

....
....
....
....

WEDNESDAY, 24

- ....
- ....
- ....
- ....

WORKOUT:

....
....
....
....

THURSDAY, 25

- ....
- ....
- ....
- ....

WORKOUT:

....
....
....
....

HAPPY + HEALTHY INTENTION:

....

WORKOUT:

- ....
- ....
- ....
- ....

WORKOUT:

- ....
- ....
- ....

WORKOUT:

- ....
- ....
- ....

Weekly Eats:

....
....
....
....
....

To Do:

....
....
....
....
....

March 2021

SUNDAY	MONDAY	TUESDAY
	1	
7	8	
14	15	1
21	22	2
28	29	3

EDNESDAY	THURSDAY	FRIDAY	SATURDAY
3	4	5	6
10	11	12	13
17	18	19	20
24	25	26	27
31			

March 2021

AT A GLANCE

March Goals:

....
....
....

March Birthdays:

....
....
....

March Anniversaries:

....
....
....

March To Do:

- ☐ ....
- ☐ ....
- ☐ ....
- ☐ ....
- ☐ ....
- ☐ ....
- ☐ ....
- ☐ ....
- ☐ ....

Habit Tracker

Habit	1	2	3	4	5	6	7	8	9	10	11	12

GRATITUDE:

SHOPPING LIST:

BUDGET:

Notes:

15	16	17	18	19	20	21	22	23	24	25	26	27	28	29	30	31

March 2021

MONDAY, 1

- ....
- ....
- ....
- ....

WORKOUT:

TUESDAY, 2

- ....
- ....
- ....
- ....

WORKOUT:

WEDNESDAY, 3

- ....
- ....
- ....
- ....

WORKOUT:

THURSDAY, 4

- ....
- ....
- ....
- ....

WORKOUT:

HAPPY + HEALTHY INTENTION:

....

FRIDAY, 5

WORKOUT:
....
....
....
....

SATURDAY, 6

WORKOUT:
....
....
....

SUNDAY, 7

WORKOUT:
....
....
....

Weekly Eats:

....
....
....
....

To Do:

....
....
....
....

March 2021

MONDAY, 8

- ....
- ....
- ....
- ....

WORKOUT:

....

....

....

....

TUESDAY, 9

- ....
- ....
- ....
- ....

WORKOUT:

....

....

....

....

WEDNESDAY, 10

- ....
- ....
- ....
- ....

WORKOUT:

....

....

....

....

THURSDAY, 11

- ....
- ....
- ....
- ....

WORKOUT:

....

....

....

....

....

....

- ....
- ....
- ....
- ....

WORKOUT:

....

....

....

....

FRIDAY, 12

- ....
- ....
- ....

WORKOUT:

....

....

....

SATURDAY, 13

- ....
- ....
- ....

WORKOUT:

....

....

....

SUNDAY, 14

Weekly Eats

....

....

....

....

....

To Do

....

....

....

....

....

March 2021

MONDAY, 15

- ....
- ....
- ....
- ....

WORKOUT:

TUESDAY, 16

- ....
- ....
- ....
- ....

WORKOUT:

WEDNESDAY, 17

- ....
- ....
- ....
- ....

WORKOUT:

THURSDAY, 18

- ....
- ....
- ....
- ....

WORKOUT:

HAPPY + HEALTHY INTENTION:

....

WORKOUT:
....
....
....
....

FRIDAY, 19

WORKOUT:
....
....
....

SATURDAY, 20

WORKOUT:
....
....
....

SUNDAY, 21

Weekly Eats:

....
....
....
....
....

To Do:

....
....
....
....
....

March 2021

MONDAY, 22

-
-
-
-

WORKOUT:

TUESDAY, 23

-
-
-
-

WORKOUT:

WEDNESDAY, 24

-
-
-
-

WORKOUT:

THURSDAY, 25

-
-
-
-

WORKOUT:

....

- ....
- ....
- ....
- ....

WORKOUT:

....
....
....

FRIDAY, 26

- ....
- ....
- ....

WORKOUT:

....
....
....

SATURDAY, 27

- ....
- ....
- ....

WORKOUT:

....
....
....

SUNDAY, 28

Weekly Eats

....
....
....
....
....

To Do

....
....
....
....
....

March 2021

MONDAY, 29

- ....
- ....
- ....
- ....

WORKOUT:

TUESDAY, 30

- ....
- ....
- ....
- ....

WORKOUT:

WEDNESDAY, 31

- ....
- ....
- ....
- ....

WORKOUT:

THURSDAY, 1

- ....
- ....
- ....
- ....

WORKOUT:

....

....

WORKOUT:

....

....

....

....

FRIDAY, 2

WORKOUT:

....

....

....

SATURDAY, 3

WORKOUT:

....

....

....

SUNDAY, 4

Weekly Eats:

....

....

....

....

....

To Do:

....

....

....

....

....

April 2021

SUNDAY	MONDAY	TUESDAY
4	5	
11	12	
18	19	2
25	26	2

WEDNESDAY	THURSDAY	FRIDAY	SATURDAY
	1	2	3
7	8	9	10
14	15	16	17
21	22	23	24
28	29	30	

April 2021

AT A GLANCE

April Goals:

....
....
....

April Birthdays:

....
....
....

April Anniversaries:

....
....
....

April To Do:

- [ ] ....
- [ ] ....
- [ ] ....
- [ ] ....
- [ ] ....
- [ ] ....
- [ ] ....
- [ ] ....
- [ ] ....

Habit Tracker

Habit	1	2	3	4	5	6	7	8	9	10	11

GRATITUDE:

SHOPPING LIST:

BUDGET:

Notes:

14	15	16	17	18	19	20	21	22	23	24	25	26	27	28	29	30

April 2021

MONDAY, 5

- ....
- ....
- ....
- ....

WORKOUT:

....
....
....
....

TUESDAY, 6

- ....
- ....
- ....
- ....

WORKOUT:

....
....
....
....

WEDNESDAY, 7

- ....
- ....
- ....
- ....

WORKOUT:

....
....
....
....

THURSDAY, 8

- ....
- ....
- ....
- ....

WORKOUT:

....
....
....
....

....

FRIDAY, 9

- ....
- ....
- ....
- ....

WORKOUT:

....
....
....

SATURDAY, 10

- ....
- ....
- ....

WORKOUT:

....
....
....

SUNDAY, 11

- ....
- ....
- ....

WORKOUT:

....
....
....

Weekly Eats:

....
....
....
....
....

To Do:

....
....
....
....
....

April 2021

MONDAY, 12

- ....
- ....
- ....
- ....

WORKOUT:

TUESDAY, 13

- ....
- ....
- ....
- ....

WORKOUT:

WEDNESDAY, 14

- ....
- ....
- ....
- ....

WORKOUT:

THURSDAY, 15

- ....
- ....
- ....
- ....

WORKOUT:

WORKOUT:

FRIDAY, 16

WORKOUT:

SATURDAY, 17

WORKOUT:

SUNDAY, 18

Weekly Eats

To Do

April 2021

MONDAY, 19

- ....
- ....
- ....
- ....

WORKOUT:

TUESDAY, 20

- ....
- ....
- ....
- ....

WORKOUT:

WEDNESDAY, 21

- ....
- ....
- ....
- ....

WORKOUT:

THURSDAY, 22

- ....
- ....
- ....
- ....

WORKOUT:

....

WORKOUT:

- ....
- ....
- ....
- ....

FRIDAY, 23

WORKOUT:

- ....
- ....
- ....
  ....

SATURDAY, 24

WORKOUT:

- ....
- ....
- ....
  ....

SUNDAY, 25

Weekly Eats:

....
....
....
....
....

To Do:

....
....
....
....
....

April 2021

MONDAY, 26

- ....
- ....
- ....
- ....

WORKOUT:

....

....

....

....

TUESDAY, 27

- ....
- ....
- ....
- ....

WORKOUT:

....

....

....

....

WEDNESDAY, 28

- ....
- ....
- ....
- ....

WORKOUT:

....

....

....

....

THURSDAY, 29

- ....
- ....
- ....
- ....

WORKOUT:

....

....

....

....

....

WORKOUT:

....

....

....

....

FRIDAY, 30

WORKOUT:

....

....

....

....

SATURDAY, 1

WORKOUT:

....

....

....

....

SUNDAY, 2

Weekly Eats

....

....

....

....

....

To Do

....

....

....

....

....

May 2021

SUNDAY	MONDAY	TUESDA
2	3	
9	10	
16	17	1
23	24	2
30	31	

EDNESDAY	THURSDAY	FRIDAY	SATURDAY
			1
5	6	7	8
12	13	14	15
19	20	21	22
26	27	28	29

May 2021

May Goals:

....
....
....

May Birthdays:

....
....
....

May Anniversaries:

....
....
....

May To Do:

☐ ....
☐ ....
☐ ....
☐ ....
☐ ....
☐ ....
☐ ....
☐ ....
☐ ....

Habit Tracker

Habit	1	2	3	4	5	6	7	8	9	10	11	12

GRATITUDE:

SHOPPING LIST:

BUDGET:

Notes:

15	16	17	18	19	20	21	22	23	24	25	26	27	28	29	30	31

May 2021

MONDAY, 3

- ....
- ....
- ....
- ....

WORKOUT:

TUESDAY, 4

- ....
- ....
- ....
- ....

WORKOUT:

WEDNESDAY, 5

- ....
- ....
- ....
- ....

WORKOUT:

THURSDAY, 6

- ....
- ....
- ....
- ....

WORKOUT:

....

- ....
- ....
- ....
- ....

WORKOUT:

....

....

....

FRIDAY, 7

- ....
- ....
- ....

WORKOUT:

....

....

....

SATURDAY, 8

- ....
- ....
- ....

WORKOUT:

....

....

....

SUNDAY, 9

Weekly Eats:

....

....

....

....

....

To Do:

....

....

....

....

....

May 2021

MONDAY, 10

WORKOUT:

TUESDAY, 11

WORKOUT:

WEDNESDAY, 12

WORKOUT:

THURSDAY, 13

WORKOUT:

HAPPY + HEALTHY INTENTION:

WORKOUT:

FRIDAY, 14

WORKOUT:

SATURDAY, 15

WORKOUT:

SUNDAY, 16

Weekly Eats

To Do

May 2021

MONDAY, 17

- ....
- ....
- ....
- ....

WORKOUT:

....
....
....
....

TUESDAY, 18

- ....
- ....
- ....
- ....

WORKOUT:

....
....
....
....

WEDNESDAY, 19

- ....
- ....
- ....
- ....

WORKOUT:

....
....
....
....

THURSDAY, 20

- ....
- ....
- ....
- ....

WORKOUT:

....
....
....
....

_____

FRIDAY, 21

WORKOUT:

- ....
- ....
- ....
- ....

SATURDAY, 22

WORKOUT:

- ....
- ....
- ....

SUNDAY, 23

WORKOUT:

- ....
- ....
- ....

Weekly Eats:

....
....
....
....
....

To Do:

....
....
....
....
....

May 2021

MONDAY, 24

- ·
- ·
- ·
- ·

WORKOUT:

TUESDAY, 25

- ·
- ·
- ·
- ·

WORKOUT:

WEDNESDAY, 26

- ·
- ·
- ·
- ·

WORKOUT:

THURSDAY, 27

- ·
- ·
- ·

WORKOUT:

HAPPY + HEALTHY INTENTION:

WORKOUT:

FRIDAY, 28

WORKOUT:

SATURDAY, 29

WORKOUT:

SUNDAY, 30

Weekly Eats:

To Do:

June 2021

SUNDAY	MONDAY	TUESDA
6	7	
13	14	
20	21	2
27	28	2

EDNESDAY	THURSDAY	FRIDAY	SATURDAY
2	3	4	5
9	10	11	12
16	17	18	19
23	24	25	26
30			

June 2021

AT A GLANCE

June Goals:

....

....

....

June Birthdays:

....

....

....

June Anniversaries:

....

....

....

June To Do:

☐ ....

☐ ....

☐ ....

☐ ....

☐ ....

....

☐ ....

....

☐ ....

....

☐ ....

....

☐ ....

....

☐ ....

Habit Tracker

Habit	1	2	3	4	5	6	7	8	9	10	11

GRATITUDE:

SHOPPING LIST:

BUDGET:

Notes:

14	15	16	17	18	19	20	21	22	23	24	25	26	27	28	29	30

June 2021

MONDAY, 31

- ....
- ....
- ....
- ....

WORKOUT:

TUESDAY, 1

- ....
- ....
- ....
- ....

WORKOUT:

WEDNESDAY, 2

- ....
- ....
- ....
- ....

WORKOUT:

THURSDAY, 3

- ....
- ....
- ....
- ....

WORKOUT:

HAPPY + HEALTHY INTENTION:

....

WORKOUT:

....

FRIDAY, 4

WORKOUT:

....

SATURDAY, 5

WORKOUT:

....

SUNDAY, 6

Weekly Eats

....

To Do

....

June 2021

MONDAY, 7

-
-
-
-

WORKOUT:

TUESDAY, 8

-
-
-
-

WORKOUT:

WEDNESDAY, 9

-
-
-
-

WORKOUT:

THURSDAY, 10

-
-
-
-

WORKOUT:

....

WORKOUT:

....

....

....

....

FRIDAY, 11

WORKOUT:

....

....

....

....

SATURDAY, 12

WORKOUT:

....

....

....

....

SUNDAY, 13

Weekly Eats:

....

....

....

....

....

To Do

....

....

....

....

....

June 2021

MONDAY, 14

-
-
-
-

WORKOUT:

TUESDAY, 15

-
-
-
-

WORKOUT:

WEDNESDAY, 16

-
-
-
-

WORKOUT:

THURSDAY, 17

-
-
-
-

WORKOUT:

....

- ....

WORKOUT:

- ....

- ....

- ....

FRIDAY, 18

WORKOUT:

- ....

- ....

- ....

SATURDAY, 19

WORKOUT:

- ....

- ....

- ....

SUNDAY, 20

Weekly Eats

....

....

....

....

....

To Do

....

....

....

....

....

June 2021

MONDAY, 21

- ....
- ....
- ....
- ....

WORKOUT:

....
....
....
....

TUESDAY, 22

- ....
- ....
- ....
- ....

WORKOUT:

....
....
....
....

WEDNESDAY, 23

- ....
- ....
- ....
- ....

WORKOUT:

....
....
....
....

THURSDAY, 24

- ....
- ....
- ....
- ....

WORKOUT:

....
....
....
....

....

WORKOUT:

....

....

....

FRIDAY, 25

....

....

....

WORKOUT:

....

....

....

SATURDAY, 26

....

....

....

WORKOUT:

....

....

....

SUNDAY, 27

Weekly Eats:

....

....

....

....

....

To Do:

....

....

....

....

....

June 2021

MONDAY, 28

-
-
-
-

WORKOUT:

TUESDAY, 29

-
-
-
-

WORKOUT:

WEDNESDAY, 30

-
-
-
-

WORKOUT:

THURSDAY, 1

-
-
-
-

WORKOUT:

HAPPY + HEALTHY INTENTION:

WORKOUT:

FRIDAY, 2

WORKOUT:

SATURDAY, 3

WORKOUT:

SUNDAY, 4

Weekly Eats

To Do

July 2021

SUNDAY	MONDAY	TUESDAY
4	5	
11	12	1
18	19	2
25	26	2

WEDNESDAY	THURSDAY	FRIDAY	SATURDAY
	1	2	3
7	8	9	10
14	15	16	17
21	22	23	24
28	29	30	31

July 2021

AT A GLANCE

July Goals:

....
....
....

July Birthdays:

....
....
....

July Anniversaries:

....
....
....

July To Do:

- ☐ ....
- ☐ ....
- ☐ ....
- ☐ ....
- ☐ ....
- ☐ ....
- ☐ ....
- ☐ ....
- ☐ ....

Habit Tracker

Habit	1	2	3	4	5	6	7	8	9	10	11	12

GRATITUDE:

SHOPPING LIST:

BUDGET:

Notes:

15	16	17	18	19	20	21	22	23	24	25	26	27	28	29	30	31

July 2021

MONDAY, 5

- ....
- ....
- ....
- ....

WORKOUT:

....
....
....
....

TUESDAY, 6

- ....
- ....
- ....
- ....

WORKOUT:

....
....
....
....

WEDNESDAY, 7

- ....
- ....
- ....
- ....

WORKOUT:

....
....
....
....

THURSDAY, 8

- ....
- ....
- ....
- ....

WORKOUT:

....
....
....
....

....

WORKOUT:

....

....

....

FRIDAY, 9

WORKOUT:

....

....

....

SATURDAY, 10

WORKOUT:

....

....

....

SUNDAY, 11

Weekly Eats:

....

....

....

....

....

To Do:

....

....

....

....

....

July 2021

MONDAY, 12

- ....
- ....
- ....
- ....

WORKOUT:

TUESDAY, 13

- ....
- ....
- ....
- ....

WORKOUT:

WEDNESDAY, 14

- ....
- ....
- ....
- ....

WORKOUT:

THURSDAY, 15

- ....
- ....
- ....
- ....

WORKOUT:

....

FRIDAY, 16

WORKOUT:

- ....
- ....
- ....
- ....

SATURDAY, 17

WORKOUT:

- ....
- ....
- ....

SUNDAY, 18

WORKOUT:

- ....
- ....
- ....

Weekly Eats

....

....

....

....

....

To Do

....

....

....

....

....

July 2021

MONDAY, 19

- ....
- ....
- ....
- ....

WORKOUT:

TUESDAY, 20

- ....
- ....
- ....
- ....

WORKOUT:

WEDNESDAY, 21

- ....
- ....
- ....
- ....

WORKOUT:

THURSDAY, 22

- ....
- ....
- ....
- ....

WORKOUT:

WORKOUT:

FRIDAY, 23

WORKOUT:

SATURDAY, 24

WORKOUT:

SUNDAY, 25

Weekly Eats:

To Do:

July 2021

MONDAY, 26

-
-
-
-

WORKOUT:

TUESDAY, 27

-
-
-
-

WORKOUT:

WEDNESDAY, 28

-
-
-
-

WORKOUT:

THURSDAY, 29

-
-
-
-

WORKOUT:

HAPPY + HEALTHY INTENTION:

....

WORKOUT:

- ....
- ....
- ....
- ....

....

FRIDAY, 30

WORKOUT:

- ....
- ....
- ....

....

SATURDAY, 31

WORKOUT:

- ....
- ....
- ....

....

SUNDAY, 1

Weekly Eats

....

....

....

....

....

To Do

....

....

....

....

....

August 2021

SUNDAY	MONDAY	TUESDAY
1	2	
8	9	1
15	16	1
22	23	2
29	30	3

WEDNESDAY	THURSDAY	FRIDAY	SATURDAY
4	5	6	7
11	12	13	14
18	19	20	21
25	26	27	28

August 2021

AT A GLANCE

August Goals:

....
....
....

August Birthdays:

....
....
....

August Anniversaries:

....
....
....

August To Do:

☐ ....
☐ ....
☐ ....
☐ ....
☐ ....
☐ ....
☐ ....
☐ ....
☐ ....

Habit Tracker

Habit	1	2	3	4	5	6	7	8	9	10	11	12

GRATITUDE:

SHOPPING LIST:

BUDGET:

Notes:

15	16	17	18	19	20	21	22	23	24	25	26	27	28	29	30	31

August 2021

MONDAY, 2

WORKOUT:

- ....
- ....
- ....
- ....

TUESDAY, 3

WORKOUT:

- ....
- ....
- ....
- ....

WEDNESDAY, 4

WORKOUT:

- ....
- ....
- ....
- ....

THURSDAY, 5

WORKOUT:

- ....
- ....
- ....
- ....

WORKOUT:

FRIDAY, 6

WORKOUT:

SATURDAY, 7

WORKOUT:

SUNDAY, 8

Weekly Eats:

To Do:

August 2021

MONDAY, 9

-
-
-
-

WORKOUT:

TUESDAY, 10

-
-
-
-

WORKOUT:

WEDNESDAY, 11

-
-
-
-

WORKOUT:

THURSDAY, 12

-
-
-
-

WORKOUT:

....

- ....
- ....
- ....
- ....

WORKOUT:

....

....

....

FRIDAY, 13

- ....
- ....
- ....

WORKOUT:

....

....

....

SATURDAY, 14

- ....
- ....
- ....

WORKOUT:

....

....

....

SUNDAY, 15

Weekly Eats

....

....

....

....

To Do

....

....

....

....

August 2021

MONDAY, 16

- ....
- ....
- ....
- ....

WORKOUT:
....
....
....
....

TUESDAY, 17

- ....
- ....
- ....
- ....

WORKOUT:
....
....
....
....

WEDNESDAY, 18

- ....
- ....
- ....
- ....

WORKOUT:
....
....
....
....

THURSDAY, 19

- ....
- ....
- ....
- ....

WORKOUT:
....
....
....
....

HAPPY + HEALTHY INTENTION:

....

WORKOUT:

....

....

....

....

FRIDAY, 20

WORKOUT:

....

....

....

SATURDAY, 21

WORKOUT:

....

....

....

SUNDAY, 22

Weekly Eats:

....

....

....

....

To Do:

....

....

....

....

....

August 2021

MONDAY, 23

- ....
- ....
- ....
- ....

WORKOUT:

TUESDAY, 24

- ....
- ....
- ....
- ....

WORKOUT:

WEDNESDAY, 25

- ....
- ....
- ....
- ....

WORKOUT:

THURSDAY, 26

- ....
- ....
- ....
- ....

WORKOUT:

HAPPY + HEALTHY INTENTION:

....

....

WORKOUT:

- ....
- ....
- ....
- ....

FRIDAY, 27

WORKOUT:

- ....
- ....
- ....

SATURDAY, 28

WORKOUT:

- ....
- ....
- ....

SUNDAY, 29

Weekly Eats:

....

....

....

....

To Do:

....

....

....

....

....

September 2021

SUNDAY	MONDAY	TUESDAY
5	6	
12	13	1
19	20	2
26	27	2

EDNESDAY	THURSDAY	FRIDAY	SATURDAY
1	2	3	4
8	9	10	11
15	16	17	18
22	23	24	25
29	30		

September 2021

AT A GLANCE

September Goals:

....
....
....

September Birthdays:

....
....
....

September Anniversaries:

....
....
....

September To Do:

- ☐ ....
- ☐ ....
- ☐ ....
- ☐ ....
- ☐ ....
- ☐ ....
- ☐ ....
- ☐ ....
- ☐ ....

Habit Tracker

Habit	1	2	3	4	5	6	7	8	9	10	11

GRATITUDE:

SHOPPING LIST:

BUDGET:

Notes:

14	15	16	17	18	19	20	21	22	23	24	25	26	27	28	29	30

September 2021

MONDAY, 30

- ....
- ....
- ....
- ....

WORKOUT:

TUESDAY, 31

- ....
- ....
- ....
- ....

WORKOUT:

WEDNESDAY, 1

- ....
- ....
- ....
- ....

WORKOUT:

THURSDAY, 2

- ....
- ....
- ....
- ....

WORKOUT:

HAPPY + HEALTHY INTENTION:

....

WORKOUT:

....

....

....

....

FRIDAY, 3

WORKOUT:

....

....

....

SATURDAY, 4

WORKOUT:

....

....

....

SUNDAY, 5

Weekly Eats

....

....

....

....

....

To Do

....

....

....

....

....

September 2021

MONDAY, 6

-
-
-
-

WORKOUT:

TUESDAY, 7

-
-
-
-

WORKOUT:

WEDNESDAY, 8

-
-
-
-

WORKOUT:

THURSDAY, 9

-
-
-
-

WORKOUT:

HAPPY + HEALTHY INTENTION:

....

- ....
- ....
- ....
- ....

WORKOUT:

....

....

....

FRIDAY, 10

- ....
- ....
- ....

WORKOUT:

....

....

....

SATURDAY, 11

- ....
- ....
- ....

WORKOUT:

....

....

....

SUNDAY, 12

Weekly Eats

....

....

....

....

....

To Do

....

....

....

....

....

September 2021

MONDAY, 13

- ....
- ....
- ....
- ....

WORKOUT:

TUESDAY, 14

- ....
- ....
- ....
- ....

WORKOUT:

WEDNESDAY, 15

- ....
- ....
- ....
- ....

WORKOUT:

THURSDAY, 16

- ....
- ....
- ....
- ....

WORKOUT:

HAPPY + HEALTHY INTENTION:

....

WORKOUT:

....

....

....

....

FRIDAY, 17

WORKOUT:

....

....

....

SATURDAY, 18

WORKOUT:

....

....

....

SUNDAY, 19

Weekly Eats:

....

....

....

....

....

To Do:

....

....

....

....

....

September 2021

MONDAY, 20

-
-
-
-

WORKOUT:

TUESDAY, 21

-
-
-
-

WORKOUT:

WEDNESDAY, 22

-
-
-
-

WORKOUT:

THURSDAY, 23

-
-
-
-

WORKOUT:

HAPPY + HEALTHY INTENTION:

....

FRIDAY, 24

WORKOUT:

- ....
- ....
- ....
- ....

SATURDAY, 25

WORKOUT:

- ....
- ....
- ....

SUNDAY, 26

WORKOUT:

- ....
- ....
- ....

Weekly Eats:

....

....

....

....

....

To Do:

....

....

....

....

....

September 2021

MONDAY, 27

- ....
- ....
- ....
- ....

WORKOUT:

TUESDAY, 28

- ....
- ....
- ....
- ....

WORKOUT:

WEDNESDAY, 29

- ....
- ....
- ....
- ....

WORKOUT:

THURSDAY, 30

- ....
- ....
- ....
- ....

WORKOUT:

HAPPY + HEALTHY INTENTION:

....

WORKOUT:

FRIDAY, 1

....

WORKOUT:

SATURDAY, 2

....

WORKOUT:

SUNDAY, 3

....

Weekly Eats

....
....
....
....
....

To Do

....
....
....
....
....

October 2021

SUNDAY	MONDAY	TUESDA
3	4	
10	11	
17	18	
24	25	
31		

EDNESDAY	THURSDAY	FRIDAY	SATURDAY
		1	2
6	7	8	9
13	14	15	16
20	21	22	23
27	28	29	30

October 2021

AT A GLANCE

October Goals:

....
....
....

October Birthdays:

....
....
....

October Anniversaries:

....
....
....

October To Do:

- ☐ ....
- ☐ ....
- ☐ ....
- ☐ ....
- ☐ ....
- ☐ ....
- ☐ ....
- ☐ ....
- ☐ ....

Habit Tracker

Habit	1	2	3	4	5	6	7	8	9	10	11	12

GRATITUDE:

SHOPPING LIST:

BUDGET:

Notes:

15	16	17	18	19	20	21	22	23	24	25	26	27	28	29	30	31

October 2021

MONDAY, 4

- ....
- ....
- ....
- ....

WORKOUT:

TUESDAY, 5

- ....
- ....
- ....
- ....

WORKOUT:

WEDNESDAY, 6

- ....
- ....
- ....
- ....

WORKOUT:

THURSDAY, 7

- ....
- ....
- ....
- ....

WORKOUT:

HAPPY + HEALTHY INTENTION:

....

	WORKOUT:	
•		**FRIDAY, 8**
•		
•		
•		

	WORKOUT:	
•		**SATURDAY, 9**
•		
•		

	WORKOUT:	
•		**SUNDAY, 10**
•		
•		

Weekly Eats

....

....

....

....

To Do

....

....

....

....

....

October 2021

MONDAY, 11

WORKOUT:

- ....
- ....
- ....
- ....

TUESDAY, 12

WORKOUT:

- ....
- ....
- ....
- ....

WEDNESDAY, 13

WORKOUT:

- ....
- ....
- ....
- ....

THURSDAY, 14

WORKOUT:

- ....
- ....
- ....
- ....

HAPPY + HEALTHY INTENTION:

WORKOUT:

FRIDAY, 15

WORKOUT:

SATURDAY, 16

WORKOUT:

SUNDAY, 17

Weekly Eats:

To Do

October 2021

MONDAY, 18

-
-
-
-

WORKOUT:

TUESDAY, 19

-
-
-
-

WORKOUT:

WEDNESDAY, 20

-
-
-
-

WORKOUT:

THURSDAY, 21

-
-
-
-

WORKOUT:

HAPPY + HEALTHY INTENTION:

....

WORKOUT:

- ....
- ....
- ....
- ....

FRIDAY, 22

WORKOUT:

- ....
- ....
- ....

SATURDAY, 23

WORKOUT:

- ....
- ....
- ....

SUNDAY, 24

Weekly Eats

....

....

....

....

....

To Do

....

....

....

....

....

October 2021

MONDAY, 25

- ....
- ....
- ....
- ....

WORKOUT:

TUESDAY, 26

- ....
- ....
- ....
- ....

WORKOUT:

WEDNESDAY, 27

- ....
- ....
- ....
- ....

WORKOUT:

THURSDAY, 28

- ....
- ....
- ....
- ....

WORKOUT:

HAPPY + HEALTHY INTENTION:

....

WORKOUT:

....

....

....

....

WORKOUT:

....

....

....

WORKOUT:

....

....

....

Weekly Eats:

....

....

....

....

....

To Do:

....

....

....

....

November 2021

SUNDAY	MONDAY	TUESDA
	1	
7	8	
14	15	
21	22	
28	29	3

WEDNESDAY	THURSDAY	FRIDAY	SATURDAY
3	4	5	6
10	11	12	13
17	18	19	20
24	25	26	27

November 2021

AT A GLANCE

November Goals:

....
....
....

November Birthdays:

....
....
....

November Anniversaries:

....
....
....

November To Do:

- [ ] ....
- [ ] ....
- [ ] ....
- [ ] ....
- [ ] ....
- [ ] ....
- [ ] ....
- [ ] ....
- [ ] ....

Habit Tracker

Habit	1	2	3	4	5	6	7	8	9	10	11

BUDGET:

Notes:

14	15	16	17	18	19	20	21	22	23	24	25	26	27	28	29	30

November 2021

MONDAY, 1

-
-
-
-

WORKOUT:

TUESDAY, 2

-
-
-
-

WORKOUT:

WEDNESDAY, 3

-
-
-
-

WORKOUT:

THURSDAY, 4

-
-
-
-

WORKOUT:

WORKOUT:

FRIDAY, 5

WORKOUT:

SATURDAY, 6

WORKOUT:

SUNDAY, 7

Weekly Eats

To Do

November 2021

MONDAY, 8

WORKOUT:

TUESDAY, 9

WORKOUT:

WEDNESDAY, 10

WORKOUT:

THURSDAY, 11

WORKOUT:

HAPPY + HEALTHY INTENTION:

....

WORKOUT:
....
....
....
....

FRIDAY, 12

WORKOUT:
....
....
....
....

SATURDAY, 13

WORKOUT:
....
....
....
....

SUNDAY, 14

Weekly Eats

....
....
....
....
....

To Do:

....
....
....
....
....

November 2021

MONDAY, 15

WORKOUT:

-
-
-
-

TUESDAY, 16

WORKOUT:

-
-
-
-

WEDNESDAY, 17

WORKOUT:

-
-
-
-

THURSDAY, 18

WORKOUT:

-
-
-
-

WORKOUT:

FRIDAY, 19

WORKOUT:

SATURDAY, 20

WORKOUT:

SUNDAY, 21

Weekly Eats:

To Do:

November 2021

WORKOUT:

WORKOUT:

WORKOUT:

WORKOUT:

WORKOUT:

FRIDAY, 26

WORKOUT:

SATURDAY, 27

WORKOUT:

SUNDAY, 28

Weekly Eats

To Do

November 2021

MONDAY, 29

-
-
-
-

WORKOUT:

TUESDAY, 30

-
-
-
-

WORKOUT:

WEDNESDAY, 1

-
-
-
-

WORKOUT:

THURSDAY, 2

-
-
-
-

WORKOUT:

HAPPY + HEALTHY INTENTION:

....

WORKOUT:

FRIDAY, 3

- ....
- ....
- ....
- ....

WORKOUT:

SATURDAY, 4

- ....
- ....
- ....

WORKOUT:

SUNDAY, 5

- ....
- ....
- ....

Weekly Eats:

....

....

....

....

....

To Do:

....

....

....

....

....

December 2021

SUNDAY	MONDAY	TUESDAY
5	6	
12	13	1
19	20	2
26	27	2

WEDNESDAY	THURSDAY	FRIDAY	SATURDAY
1	2	3	4
8	9	10	11
15	16	17	18
22	23	24	25
29	30	31	

December 2021

AT A GLANCE

December Goals:

....
....
....

December Birthdays:

....
....
....

December Anniversaries:

....
....
....

December To Do:

- [ ] ....
- [ ] ....
- [ ] ....
- [ ] ....
- [ ] ....
- [ ] ....
- [ ] ....
- [ ] ....
- [ ] ....

Habit Tracker

Habit	1	2	3	4	5	6	7	8	9	10	11	12

GRATITUDE:

SHOPPING LIST:

BUDGET:

Notes:

15	16	17	18	19	20	21	22	23	24	25	26	27	28	29	30	31

December 2021

MONDAY, 6

WORKOUT:

TUESDAY, 7

WORKOUT:

WEDNESDAY, 8

WORKOUT:

THURSDAY, 9

WORKOUT:

WORKOUT:

FRIDAY, 10

WORKOUT:

SATURDAY, 11

WORKOUT:

SUNDAY, 12

Weekly Eats

To Do

December 2021

MONDAY, 13

-
-
-
-

WORKOUT:

TUESDAY, 14

-
-
-
-

WORKOUT:

WEDNESDAY, 15

-
-
-
-

WORKOUT:

THURSDAY, 16

-
-
-
-

WORKOUT:

HAPPY + HEALTHY INTENTION:

WORKOUT:

FRIDAY, 17

WORKOUT:

SATURDAY, 18

WORKOUT:

SUNDAY, 19

Weekly Eats

To Do

December 2021

MONDAY, 20

- ....
- ....
- ....
- ....

WORKOUT:

....
....
....

TUESDAY, 21

- ....
- ....
- ....
- ....

WORKOUT:

....
....
....

WEDNESDAY, 22

- ....
- ....
- ....
- ....

WORKOUT:

....
....
....

THURSDAY, 23

- ....
- ....
- ....
- ....

WORKOUT:

....
....
....

FRIDAY, 24

WORKOUT:

SATURDAY, 25

WORKOUT:

SUNDAY, 26

WORKOUT:

Weekly Eats

To Do

December 2021

MONDAY, 27

-
-
-
-

WORKOUT:

TUESDAY, 28

-
-
-
-

WORKOUT:

WEDNESDAY, 29

-
-
-
-

WORKOUT:

THURSDAY, 30

-
-
-
-

WORKOUT:

....

WORKOUT:

- ....
- ....
- ....
- ....

FRIDAY, 31

WORKOUT:

- ....
- ....
- ....

SATURDAY, 1

WORKOUT:

- ....
- ....
- ....

SUNDAY, 2

Weekly Eats:

....

....

....

....

....

To Do:

....

....

....

....

....

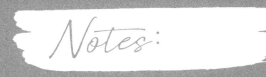

Notes:

Notes:

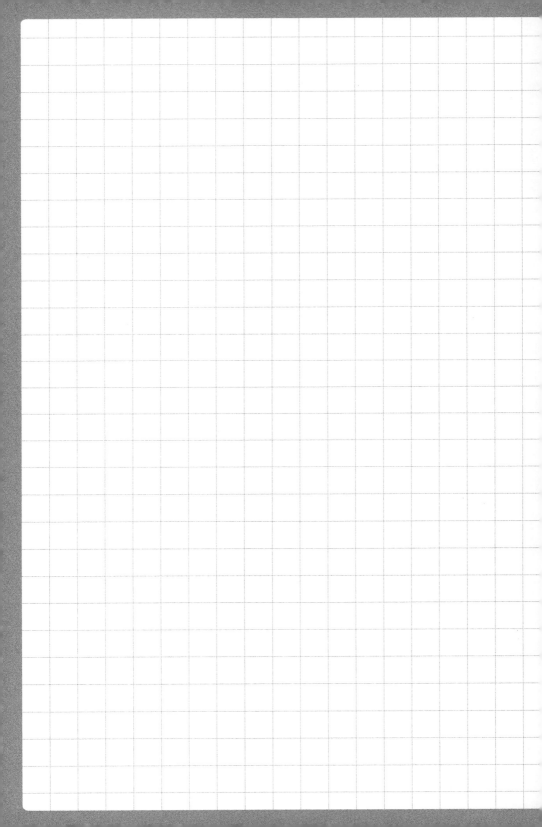

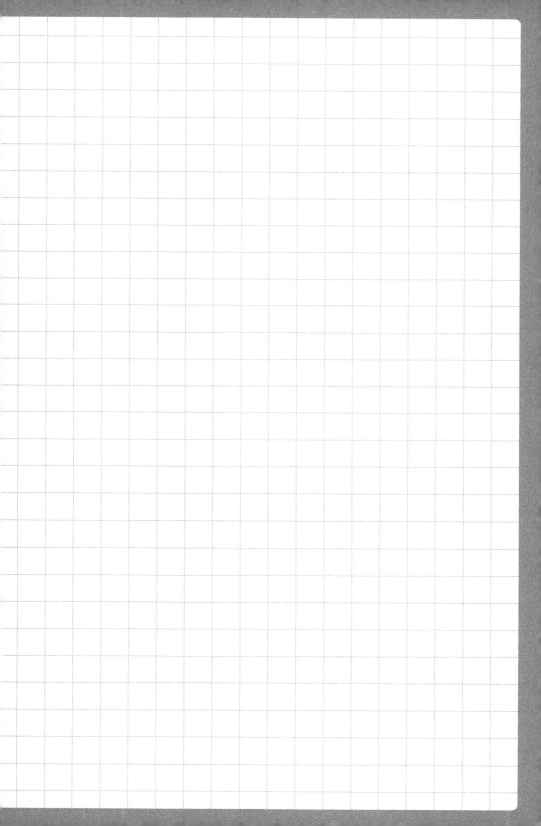

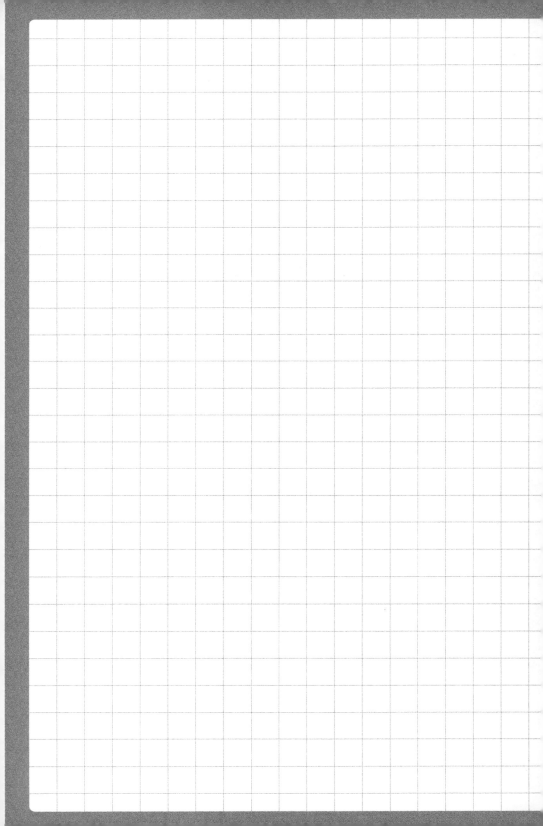

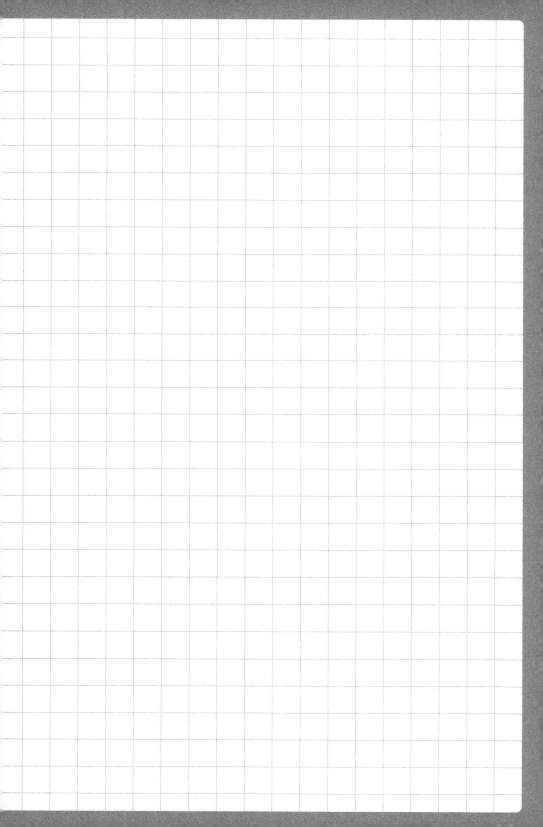

CPSIA information can be obtained
at www.ICGtesting.com
Printed in the USA
LVHW070608190121
676860LV00007B/320